WHERE INTIMACY BEGINS

THE WORKBOOK

CJ GRACELYN RAE

outskirts press

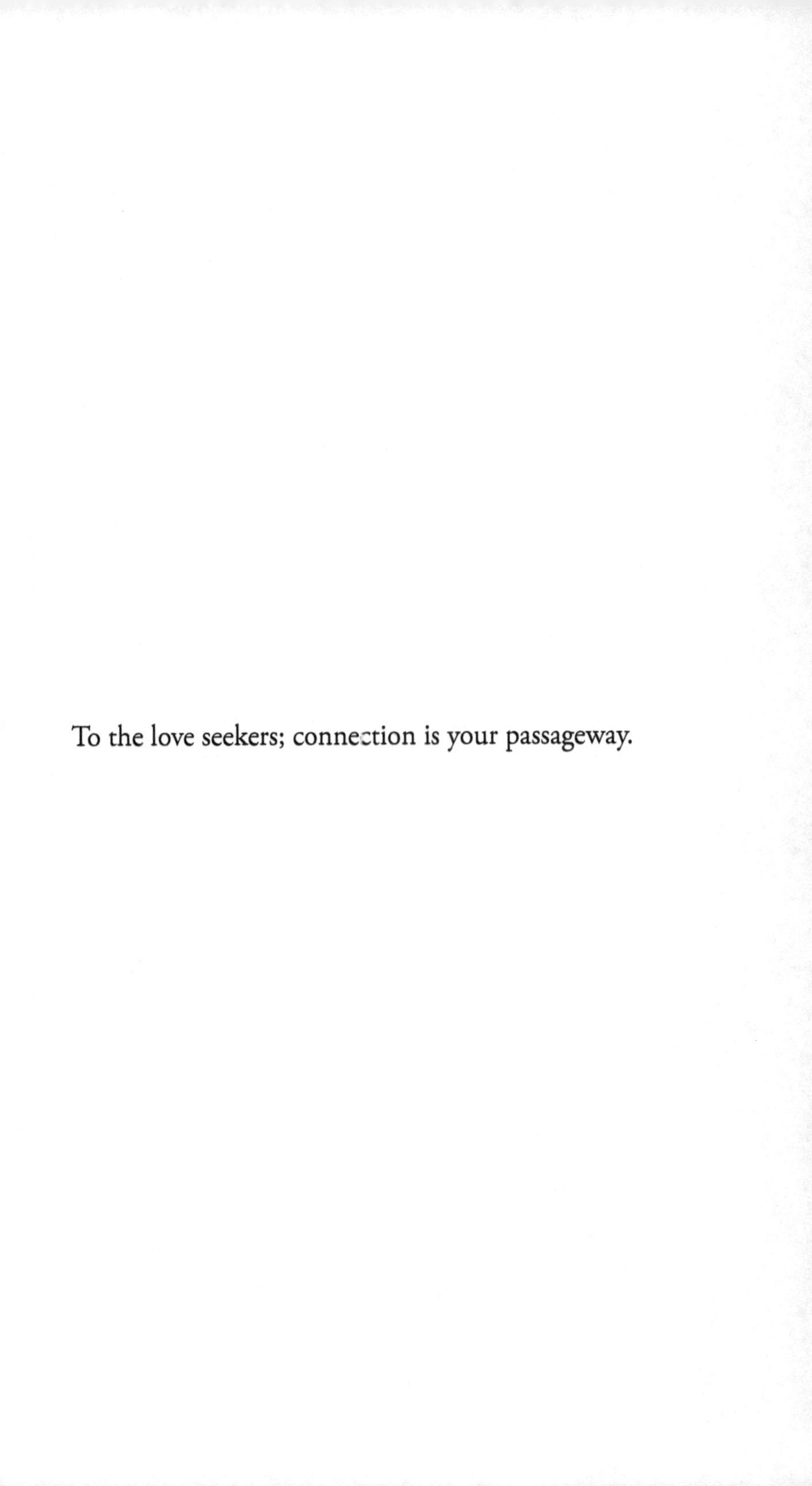

To the love seekers; connection is your passageway.

A Message from the Founders

The journey of *Where Intimacy Begins: The Workbook* and The Bonded Box* began after a group of four friends decided to bring awareness to the desire for closer bonds and intimacy in their relationships. Many women and men find the intimate connection with their partners lessens as their relationships age. Oftentimes people struggle to discuss this openly, and therapy can feel forced or uncomfortable. For some, it feels like failure of themselves, their relationship, or their marriage. In reality, many factors lead to the erosion of intimacy. These include the burden of work, intensive parenting, social pressure, financial stress, and overuse of technology, to name a few.

Intimacy is a feeling of physical and emotional closeness that is fostered by creating a deep connection with yourself or another person. This does not always need to be about lengthy discussions. It does not always have to be about sex. There is no one size fits all for intimacy. It is about finding what works for you as an individual and as a couple.

We are passionate about connection and believe in the bonds that we share with those we love. While there are no guarantees, our goal is to help couples enhance intimacy through a fun and whimsical experience. Whether you are new on this journey or an experienced traveler, we want this to be enjoyable for everyone.

We encourage you to be vulnerable as you reflect on your relationships. Take a deep breath, relax, and open your mind. Remember not to take yourself or your partner too seriously in this process, and be forgiving of any missteps that take place. "Practice makes perfect" definitely applies to learning how to communicate and please each other in the bedroom. And just a reminder, this is not Hollywood so it's never going to be perfect, but it can be great.

Our intention is to guide you into a stronger and more intimate relationship with yourself and your partner. In the following pages, we will provide you with an introduction to intimacy through the many stages of connection. We understand that reading excerpts on intimacy may not be for everyone, but if given the chance, this workbook will provide you with beneficial information about learning to connect better in and out of the bedroom. For some, getting to the contents of the box and into your birthday suits may be far more exciting than reading, so we wanted to give you a quick guide too. Our Cliff Notes version is provided at the back of *Where Intimacy Begins: The*

Workbook. Feel free to skip the frills and read Appendix A: The Great Climax. We hope you enjoy taking this journey with us and are rewarded with a fulfilling relationship with yourself and your romantic partner.

Wishing you light, love, and laughter in this endeavor.

*If you have not experienced The Bonded Box intimacy kits, you may order these thrilling activities for yourself or to share with your partner at TheBondedBox.com.

The Journey

Self-Love

The most important relationship you will ever have is with yourself. A strong, healthy, and intimate relationship starts from within. It is beneficial to take a step back from the external stressors that occupy your mind and take a moment to connect with your inner self. This gives your mind, body, and spirit the time they need to re energize and heal. Once you're happy, confident, and compassionate with yourself, you will be more apt to attract and sustain a healthy relationship with another if you so choose.

Self-esteem is the confidence you have in your personal worth and abilities. These beliefs affect how much love you are able to give and receive in your relationships. Positive self-esteem is associated with improved mental health, healthier partnerships, and more successful outcomes socially and professionally. Conversely, a lack of confidence can create feelings of self-doubt and insecurity. These concerns may surface in the midst of relationships and can interrupt the intimate connection. Overemphasizing the importance of superficial traits, as mainstream media does, can impact how you see yourself; try not to compare yourself to others. Knowing you are "good enough" is important, and incorporating self-worth building activities can be helpful.

TIPS FOR SELF-CARE

1. **Take charge.** You are in control of your life. Your choices matter. Your courage and strength will grow with this realization.
2. **Think positively.** Your thoughts create your reality. Focus on the good things and practice gratitude.
3. **Choose you.** Check in with yourself. Make positive changes for self-growth. Realize that you are worthy. Fill your own cup rather than depending on another to fill it for you.
4. **Be strong.** Challenges and obstacles that life has thrown at you over the years will one day make you stronger. Reflection provides wisdom, and resiliency comes with time.
5. **Maintain perspective.** Approach things with a positive attitude. Treat every experience as a lesson to grow from. *We cannot change the cards we are dealt, just how we play the hand* (Randy Pausch, *The Last Lecture.* Hyperion, 2008).
6. **Remember that it's never too late.** It's never too late to dream or to discover a new passion. It's never too

late to believe in new beginnings, start over, and make beautiful new memories.

SOUL-STRENGTHENING EXERCISES

- **Get moving.** Exercise is an amazing way to build your self-confidence and increase your strength both mentally and physically. Endorphins (the feel good hormones) are released during exercise and can greatly improve your mood.
  » Running, walking, weight lifting, cycling, yoga, etc. are all excellent strength-building and confidence-boosting activities.
- **Read self-help books.** These come in a variety of topics and have many benefits, including finding a solution to a problem that you may be experiencing, increasing clarity and focus when you're feeling overwhelmed, and opening your mind to new approaches when feeling stuck.
- **Practice positive self-talk.** Implementing this powerful practice regularly can boost confidence, motivation, and productivity.
- **Listen to personal growth and motivational podcasts.** Podcasts are a great way to learn something new and practice active listening.
  » Try listening to a meditation podcast to increase mindfulness by exploring feelings and gaining an understanding of thoughts.
- **Journal.** Record your feelings with the optional use of guided questions and prompts for self-discovery to help process emotions, reduce stress, and learn about yourself.

- **Get comfortable with your body.** Love your physical form and tell yourself how sexy you are when you look in the mirror. Explore what feels good for you.
    » Take a bath, light candles, and put on some relaxing music. Touch yourself in a sensual manner in sensual places. Use toys and be exploratory, creative, and sexually open with yourself.

CONFIDENCE-BUILDING ACTIVITY

Write down the name of one or two people you admire. Now record multiple characteristics of those people (it's okay if they repeat). For example: courageous, bold, empathetic, loving, gracious, resourceful, powerful, confident, and/or resilient—whatever it is that you find appealing.

Now use some of these characteristics and start describing yourself. Be kind. Write down everything you love about yourself. Remind yourself daily of these traits.

Creating intimacy starts with self-worth. When you feel confident, you are free to give and receive love on a deeper level. Now is the time to take action and truly embrace your own inner and outer beauty. Unapologetically love yourself!

Additional confidence-building activities are available in **Appendix B: Emotional Intimacy.**

LEARN TO LISTEN

Communication is the foundation of your connection with your partner. Successful communication involves active listening, sharing your feelings, and empathizing. Learning to communicate well helps you to share your needs and desires. It also allows you to reveal vulnerabilities and express empathy. When sharing with your partner, it is important to feel heard and also to listen. The ultimate goal here is to help you feel more connected in and out of the sheets, so let's get going.

Most people are guilty of half listening in conversations while they are trying to multitask work and home duties, texting on their phone, or watching TV. Think about it: when was the last time you weren't doing other tasks or had your phone nearby while your partner was trying to talk to you? Over time, your partner may not feel valued due to these repeated distractions.

It is important to actively listen to your partner to strengthen emotional intimacy.

Tips for Active Listening

- **Be present.** Be in close proximity with your partner and maintain eye contact.
- **Minimize negative body language.** Sighs and eye-rolling are counterproductive.
- **Limit interruptions.** Be patient. Allow your partner to finish their thoughts. Take turns.
- **Hear your partner.** Listen and process with intention and thoughtfulness.
- **Respond with care.** Your words matter. Repeat or re-phrase what your partner shared with you to show that you were listening. Offer feedback and support with empathy.
- **Provide a judgment free zone.** Give your partner a safe space to express themselves.
- **Stay calm.** Overreaction and/or negativity can lead to shutdown.
- **Be open.** Be willing to compromise ideas, offer solutions if necessary, and accept advice.

Active listening takes time to develop and gets rusty if not practiced. Relearning to communicate can feel awkward after a period of disconnection. Be patient and kind if you find yourself in this situation. It gets much easier with time and practice, and will eventually be spontaneous rather than forced. You are on the path to a deeper, more meaningful connection.

1. Plan a time when you both can feel comfortable and vulnerable.
2. Be sure to minimize distractions before you begin (silence your phone).
3. Engage in a conversation. Pick a topic you are interested in (take turns choosing).
4. Repeat what is being said periodically. This shows that you are following the conversation and that you are actively listening.
5. Detect their tone and pay attention to the nonverbal cues they give you. Nod, smile, give some type of nonverbal acknowledgement that you are engaged.
6. Ask questions about things you find interesting. Ask about feelings and responses. Inquire about the setting or persons involved. Show you care by being involved in the discussion.

Keep trying this exercise with new topics that are both serious and fun. Practicing these techniques will improve your overall communication. Remember to be positive. The goal is to keep the conversation flowing.

Healthy communication is important for the growth of any relationship and key for intimate bonding. Sharing your feelings and opinions with your partner will help you gain insight on their personal values, which will lead to a better understanding of each other. Continue to express your feelings and listen to your partner. Try not to take your conversations for granted. Start fresh and give your next exchange the chance to really inspire you both.

Stage 3

TIME WELL SPENT

Second to communication in improving intimacy is dedicating quality time to your partner. This means attention without outside disruptions. Thoughtfully spending your time together without distractions will continue to strengthen your connection.

It is important for every healthy relationship to carve out quality time for each other. You may be busy with work, household chores, child-rearing or hobbies, and not taking designated time for your partner. You may be kissing them goodbye as you run out the door, and kissing them goodnight after a long day, but find yourselves spending little to no time intimately connecting. Unfortunately, the close proximity of partners leans into taking their presence for granted. Prioritizing quality time is a must, and this starts with a conversation followed by effort and implementation.

So How Do You Do This?

1. **Plan.** Set dates and make it routine; Saturday night is date night. Take turns choosing to include interests you both enjoy. If you have children together, this means finding childcare options for your date nights. Quality time as a family is very important, but finding time for just the two of you is essential in building and sustaining intimacy.
2. **Turn off devices for tech-free time together.** Television can be an exception for a fun movie date night while cuddling on the couch or in bed.
3. **Try something new together.** Get creative; go to an art class or try rock climbing. If you have children, include them in your planned adventures occasionally. Witnessing your partner experience joy with your children by working as a team and bonding as a family can bring a couple closer together.
4. **Do routine things together.** Go to the gym or cook together. Household chores can also be a bonding experience and free up time for preferred activities.
5. **Be present and actively listen to your partner.** Refer back to Stage 2.
6. **Staycation.** Book a local hotel and make dinner plans at a restaurant. Being outside of the home can make the experience feel fresh and new.

Ultimately, everyone wants to feel connected. Take time tonight, turn off your cell phone, and talk to the one you love. Your partner is waiting and looking forward to spending quality time with you. Open those calendars and mark those dates.

Stage 4

TRUST AND KINDNESS

To trust or not to trust? Let your instincts be your guide. It could be argued that the most important aspect of intimacy is trust, and trust cannot be built without kindness. Consistently warm and affectionate behavior lends a much more trusting connection. On the other hand, unpleasantness and lack of loyalty leads to the fall of relationships—a reminder to be conscious of how you interact with your partner. The secret to unconditional love is trust and kindness.

What comes to mind when you think of trust? Some people may think of "cheating" when the word "trust" is mentioned, but developing a trusting relationship that promotes intimacy is much bigger than focusing on one's level of faithfulness to their partner. Trust is the ability to rely on your partner with your feelings and vulnerabilities because you feel comfortable and safe in their presence. Listening to and supporting each other, showing consideration, and having mutual respect are examples of trust. Trusting someone with your heart is sacred and should be taken seriously. It takes time to develop and requires ongoing effort to maintain, but it is necessary to establish the intimate connection you desire.

TRUST-BUILDING GUIDANCE

1. **Trust yourself first.** Trust your intuition or inner voice. Be confident in your decisions and how you feel in a situation. Be open with your vulnerabilities when the time is right, and pay attention to early red flags.
2. **Challenge negative thinking.** This is especially true if you are new to a relationship; however, give your partner the benefit of the doubt. Don't let the negative experiences from previous relationships affect your ability to trust again.
3. **Actions speak louder than words.** Make sure what you say is meaningful, and follow through on what you say. Be mindful of this in your actions, but also observe your partner's behavior and communicate inconsistencies.
4. **Be vulnerable.** Allow yourself to be emotionally available with authenticity by being honest and open.
5. **Respect.** Everyone likes to be treated well, so be kind. Honor your partner by being considerate of their feelings.
6. **Negotiate and bend.** When you're willing to give for the comfort of your partner, it sends a clear message that their needs matter to you. Compromise and sacrifice are essential when developing a higher level of trust.

Trust-Building Exercise

Take some time to ask your partner the following questions and discuss their answers together. Be sure both partners get a chance to ask and answer each question.

1. What do trust and commitment mean to you?
2. What do you need from me to show that I am committed to our relationship?
3. When you are upset, how would you like me to respond to help you?
4. What brings you joy and happiness?
5. Do you think it is acceptable to keep things from each other?

Everyone wants to feel secure and confident, not only in themselves but also with their partners. Building a trusting relationship will help foster your intimacy and make it last. Take your time and allow your new trusting journey to begin.

THE LANGUAGE OF LOVE

You may have heard of the five love languages. Just as there are different spoken languages used to communicate, there are also different languages in love. These can be helpful to identify when connecting with your partner. Love languages describe the different ways people feel loved and appreciated. Being able to decode this will help in understanding yourself and forming a deeper intimate connection with your partner.

First, you want to recognize what gets your engine going and do those things for yourself. A reminder that self-love is the first love. This will also take the pressure off your partner, in turn, allowing your partner to be more appreciated for what they can bring to the relationship.

It is equally important to understand your partner's love language while identifying your own. This is not some complicated code you have to crack alone. Communicate your needs to one another. When reviewing the different love languages, most people find that they relate to one specifically, while others resonate with a combination of more than one love language. Discover what speaks to you and share that with your partner. The information in the table below was adapted from Gary Chapman's book, *The Five Love Languages* (Northfield Publishing, 1992).

Table 1: Love Language Description and Actions

Love Language	Description	Actions
Words of Affirmation	This is where your partner requires praise from you.	Give compliments. Acknowledge their efforts. Tell your partner what you respect about them. Provide positive communication..
Acts of Service	Show thoughtful and supportive acts that your partner would appreciate.	Cook your partner a surprise meal. Do extra household chores. Take over child-rearing duties for the day if you have children. Clean their car and fill the gas tank.
Receiving Gifts	This is when your partner appreciates receiving tangible gifts.	Bring home flowers for your partner. Buy or make them a heartfelt card or leave a love note. Gift what you know they like. Give without expecting a gift in return.
Quality Time	The gift of time is precious. Be sure to make and spend quality time with your partner.	Give your undivided attention during conversations. Go for a walk. Play a card/board game Plan a date or vacation. Put your phones away and just be with one another.
Physical Touch	Your partner prefers physical actions of love over other expressions.	Hold hands. Kiss. Cuddle on the couch. Massage each other. Make time for foreplay and sex.

While these love languages have been around for several decades, there has been new research identifying seven modern love styles. Five of these styles are very similar to the above love languages; however, we are highlighting two new love styles below that are important and beneficial to developing intimacy.

Table 2: Love Style Description and Actions

Love Style	Description	Actions
Emotional	Be present for the emotional highs and lows of a relationship.	Connect and support your partner through happiness, sadness, fear, and hope. Provide a safe space for your partner to share their feelings.
Intellectual	Connect through the mind.	Value your partner's intelligence. Respect each other's opinions. Take part in thoughtful discussion of important issues.

Emotional and intellectual stimulation can lead to gratifying intimate experiences. Practice expressing love in the style that your partner craves. Be open and encourage one another. Sharing your confirmed love language/style is a great way to learn something new about each other and further enhance your connection. Your partner will feel connected if you take the time to learn and show them love in the specific way they best receive it.

 WHERE INTIMACY BEGINS

Love Language/Style Challenge

1. Separately write down on paper what your primary love language and/or style is.
2. List three related activities your partner could do for you that you would enjoy.
3. On the same piece of paper, write what you think your partner's love language is.
4. Write three actions you could do for your partner that you think they would appreciate.
5. Share your writings with each other and pay close attention to what they share.
6. Try to put these suggestions into action as early as possible.
7. Repeat this challenge with another love language/style if you have more than one.

Remember, not everyone has the same love language/style or communicates in the same way. Sometimes it takes a little time to learn what works for both you and your partner. Be mindful that you may not always get it quite right, but the act of trying is worth its own recognition and appreciation. Gratitude for efforts given will also help elevate the connection with your partner.

Learning to speak and understand the love languages/styles that are important in your relationship can deepen your romantic connection. So, which are you? Which is your partner? Take the time to find out. It will be worth it.

Stage 6

OPENNESS IS KEY

Emotional openness in a relationship is the ability to reveal one's inner thoughts and feelings, and is cultivated by healthy communication, trust building, and kindness. It also primes the foundation for a physical openness that is not only fun, but also more rewarding in the pleasure department. Don't be afraid to disclose the more personal aspects of yourself to your partner as those deeper feelings are important for them to understand. When you feel emotionally open and connected with your partner, it is much easier to be open-minded and comfortable in the bedroom.

Physical openness is a willingness to approach romantic physical connection without preconceived ideas or judgment. Being open can be challenging, especially when feeling a little nervous about what is being presented, but it can also be exciting. Those who have a tendency to put their guard up may find it difficult to participate. Undressing in front of your partner, having sex with the lights on, or experimenting with adult toys are all examples of physical openness. Remember to be patient with yourself and your partner. Awareness is key, and working through your challenges provides for growth and a stronger bond. This is an opportunity to try something new or learn something deeper about your partner or yourself, and can lead to a more fulfilling sexual connection.

How-Tos of Emotional and Physical Openness

1. **Be encouraging and make it safe:** You want your partner to share their interests with you without judgment.
2. **Respect boundaries:** Clearly communicate your boundaries with your partner. It is okay to say no if you are not comfortable with a proposition.
3. **Lean into curiosity:** Challenge yourself and your partner. Research and create a new adventure. This is where the fun can really happen.
4. **Compromise and be creative in the bedroom:** This can be done with your partner in a healthy way to show that you are open to new ideas.
5. **Ideas for physical openness include the following:**
   a. Try new ways of physically connecting to your partner without sex: massage, shaving each other, taking a bath together, washing their hair, applying lotion to their body.
   b. Try new sexual positions if you're physically connecting through sex (see Stage 10).

c. Share sex stories with friends/partners to encourage new ideas.

d. Experiment with toys and oils.

e. Masturbate alone or in front of your partner, allowing them to watch you orgasm.

f. Role play (check out role-play ideas in Stage 7).

g. Record your session/take photos.

h. Engage in oral sex. Ask your partner how they like it.

i. Talk "dirty" to each other.

j. Watch porn together. (It's important to note, if one partner is watching porn alone frequently, it can interfere with the intimacy of the couple and become a barrier for connection. Honest communication regarding this as a couple is helpful.)

ACTIVITY FOR ROMANTIC NONSEXUAL PHYSICAL CONNECTION

"Breathe Each Other" Technique

1. Stand, sit, or lie next to each other in a comfortable position.

2. Gently put your faces together with your mouths slightly open.

3. Slowly and rhythmically breathe long breaths together. One person inhales while the other exhales.

4. Fall into the comfort of being close together while connecting on a physical level.

5. This breathing technique creates a flow of energy, strengthening your intimate connection.

With intimacy there is a repetitive theme to be open, honest, and willing to communicate effectively. Be patient and offer support to one another as you continue to bond. If you see that one of you is struggling with emotional or physical openness, acknowledge the moment and work through it together. Couples with higher levels of intimacy are great communicators and have more satisfaction in both their emotional and physical connections. The effort put in will certainly pay off, and your relationship will thank you.

ADULTS PLAY TOO

Play, both sexual and nonsexual, is a great way to enrich your relationship. The personalized experience of play can help couples to develop their sense of security, improve communication, and bring special meaning to the connection. Having fun helps to release endorphins…the happy hormones. Shared happiness improves relationship satisfaction and enhances intimacy.

Play is a mindset. Couples spend a significant amount of time having fun when they first start dating. After being together for a while, it's a common report that they don't make as much time for fun. If you have lost the ability to connect in this way, it's helpful to remember that play is about being flexible, spontaneous, and open with your partner in new ways. This is a reminder that the attitude about having fun needs to be encouraged and nurtured together. Be silly and creative when exploring options; fostering laughter and lightheartedness strengthens bonds and makes resolving conflict easier for couples.

Fun Activities for Connection

Dance to your favorite songs and sing out loud.

Talk to each other in a different accent (or try).

Flirt and give each other nicknames.

Tease each other and share inside jokes. Laughter is good medicine.

Watch and/or make playful videos together at your comfort level.

Play truth or dare. Enjoy learning new things about each other and get a little wild.

Play cards or an interactive board game. Place sex acts as wagers for the winner of the game, or play naked Twister.

Go skinny-dipping.

Role-play.

One of the most thrilling ways a couple can connect is using sexual role-play. Role-play can increase excitement and enhance eroticism between you and your partner. It is helpful in reducing sexual inhibitions and allows you to indulge in fantasies or fetishes you may not be comfortable exploring otherwise.

Guide for Role-Play

1. **Set boundaries:** Discuss fantasies/fetishes you are interested in, what you are open to trying and ideas that are out. Also, understand safe practices and consider adding a safe word if trying out dominance and submission (Ds) to ensure that everyone stays in a safe space. Consider making a Yes/No/Maybe list of ideas you are interested in exploring. Be direct and honest.

2. **Decide on what to role play:** Talk about it. Do you want to take on a character or alter ego? What setting do you want to be in? Do you need props? Do you have the clothing/costumes you want to wear? What roles are you going to take on (submissive versus dominant)?

3. **Don't stress:** This is fun. Remove pressure and expectations. Don't be afraid to really act and take on the character. It's okay if you feel silly doing it. Don't judge. Be supportive.

4. **Start small and build:** Keep it simple and build on the skills you learn and things you enjoy. Continue to have ongoing conversations about what you like and don't like.

Role-Play Ideas

Strangers in a hotel bar

Pilot and flight attendant

Massage therapist and client

Nurse and adult patient

   WHERE INTIMACY BEGINS

The following vignette can be appealing for both beginners and veterans when experimenting with this playful activity. Role-play is very personal; don't be afraid to share your desires with your partner and dive into your fantasies.

Stranger in the Room

She was sitting there, legs open without any panties on, wearing a tight, red, strapless barely there dress covering her breasts and midsection. She turned her head and stared straight at him. She slipped off her bar stool and started walking his way.

Her piercing eyes never blinked or lost connection with his. Her long, thick, glistening hair bounced, as her breasts did, as she strode toward him.

He was wearing a suit from work, thinly lined, and his erection could be seen. He knew she could see it.

She put her perfectly manicured hand on his shoulder and whispered in his ear, "Are you going to fuck me on our kitchen counter or what, Handsome?"

He was taken back. He had no idea his wife had such an independent, assertive, and powerful persona (plus the wig and fake eyelashes) lingering in her bones.

Revisit some of the fun activities you used to do as a couple early in the relationship. Continue to do things that you enjoy now. Plan fun activities for your future. Dive back into laughing together and enjoy the bond you continue to strengthen.

People don't stop playing because they grow old. They grow old when they forget to play (George Bernard Shaw).

Additional fun inspiration and role-play ideas are available to you in **Appendix E: Play Activities.**

Stage 8

❧

Ignite Your Senses

On this journey, it is also helpful to learn, absorb, and practice the skills necessary to open up your relationship for the next level of play: the sensory experience. You have the power to unleash a raw and stimulating experience that can elevate your connection to a higher level simply by utilizing your five senses. Touch, taste, smell, sight, and hearing are gifts individuals use on a daily basis, but when exercised thoughtfully in the bedroom, it can be a game changer.

With life and its duties, people seldom embrace the intricacies and interactions of the day. Can you recall the last time you were actually living and feeling the moment, just you with your five senses? This is your reminder to slow it down. No matter what phase of a relationship you are in, exploring your senses is a fun way to connect with your partner. The goal is to learn more about your partner's mind and body through intimate and erotic touch and play, heightening your sexual experiences.

Challenge yourself and your partner to enjoy each other's body by engaging the five senses. Use your imagination and develop a sensory plan to help you experience your partner on this deeper level. Experiment and test each other's physical and mental thresholds. Touch, taste, smell, and see every crevice of your partner's body while actively listening for their pleasure cues. Make a deliberate attempt to try to tantalize every one of the senses. Take some time and explore the following activity for an intoxicating sensory experience.

ACTIVITY FOR IGNITING YOUR SENSES

1. **Tap into taste:** Taste your partner's body. Kiss them, and enjoy flavored lube or even lollipops by running them up and down their body or pleasure spots. You can incorporate honey, fruit, chocolate, and whipped cream—whatever the mood brings. Take a sip of your favorite drink and let it drip out of your mouth and into your partner's. Incorporate taste into your foreplay and sex.

2. **Tap into touch:** The skin is the biggest organ of our bodies. It is able to detect temperature, texture, and wetness. Use a tickler and run it up and down your partner's body. Use ice and tease your partner by running it over areas of arousal. Dildo usage is prime time for a sensory experience. Change the vibration or the depth of penetration. Blindfold your partner to intensify the touch experience.

3. **Tap into smell:** Light a candle and create the mood. You can wear your partner's favorite scent and tap into their olfactory centers. Utilize scented massage oils. Go in between your partner's legs and explore each other's smells. Those special scents are the best aphrodisiac.

4. **Tap into sight:** Use a candle to create a warm and sensual experience. Use lingerie and the art of seduction. Striptease and erotic dance can be incorporated. Mutual masturbation is highly erotic. Gaze into each other's eyes while erotically touching each other.

5. **Tap into hearing:** Set the mood with background music. You can choose naughty "fuck me" music or sensual, soft love-making music. The music helps create the mood. You can use the rhythm of the music to pace your stroke. Whisper into your lover's ear. Let yourself go, moan, and grunt in moments of pleasure.

Utilizing the five senses plays a key role in sexual arousal. When done well it can yield toe-curling physical pleasure and improve your overall intimate connection. Most importantly, heightening your sensory experience leads to the creation of core memories, strengthening your bond.

Stage 9

—⁂—

EXPLORING ORAL

Foreplay is a key component of a healthy sexual relationship, and oral sex can be an exciting and important part of it. Oral sex shows your partner that you care about their pleasure, and it can increase the intimacy and closeness you share. This intimate act can be quite arousing and should be fun for both the giver and receiver.

Some couples don't just jump right into sexual intercourse. Your body needs to warm up and your mind needs to be free from stress. Oral sex can help to relax and arouse your mind and body in order to get in the mood to accept pleasure and potentially improve the sexual experience. Be open to sharing with your partner what your comfort level is in both giving and receiving oral sex.

Suggestions for the giver to inspire you to put your skills where your mouth is:

1. Use your senses. Look at your partner's beautiful parts and take it all in. Use your hands and your breath. Slowly and gently begin to run your fingers and hands over your partner's genitalia. If your partner is female, begin by softly touching her thighs and gently moving your fingers upward toward her labia. If your partner is male, try gliding your hand over the shaft and down to the scrotum. Softly explore the entire area with your fingers, your hands, and your warm breath.

2. Take your time. You and your partner will most likely be showing a great deal of arousal at this point. Notice what is happening. Is your partner showing signs of pleasure? Are they moving, moaning, and/or breathing heavily? Is it turning you on? Pay attention to how you are both responding and this can serve as a guide to move you both toward more pleasure. If receiving, do not be afraid to give gentle hints or clues to what you like and don't like through body language and verbal communication.

3. Use your tongue and your lips. Slowly and gently start to use your mouth on and around your partner's genitalia. Be willing to explore and dive in with all parts of your mouth, but remember to take it slow at first and pay attention to your partner's body language. The slightest flick of the tongue or soft warm kiss with your lips can elicit extreme pleasure for the person receiving.

4. If performing oral sex on a woman (cunnilingus), try softly licking and touching around her labia and clitoris. Softly circling the outside parts of her clit can be extremely arousing and at times can even bring her to climax. Be gentle at first, but feel free to increase pressure and speed if that is what your partner wants. You may even want to insert a finger or vibrator into her vagina and/or anus to increase intensity and pleasure at the time of climax. If performing on a man (fellatio), try licking and touching the length of his shaft and scrotum. Use your tongue and your lips lightly at first. Play around and make sure he is ready for you to take his entirety into your mouth. Lightly suck and kiss the tip of his penis and down the length of his shaft. Read his body language to help guide you into what is most pleasurable. Anal stimulation during climax for a male can also be very pleasurable. Ask your partner what their comfort level is before trying new techniques.

5. Use your words. Communicate in order to find out their desires. Ask your partner if they are enjoying what you are doing. Ask if they prefer you to slow down, speed up, move to a different area, or keep doing what you are doing. Don't be afraid to ask, "Do you like that?" It can be very arousing, and most people are happy to engage with a partner who is so considerate and attentive to their needs.

6. Explore different positions. There are several positions that can be explored when performing oral sex. These positions depend on your mood, comfort level, creativity, and agility. We have provided a few oral sex

positions on the following page as inspiration if you and your partner are open to exploring.

7. Oral sex does not always have to end in climax. In fact, many people use oral sex as a form of foreplay to get their partner in the mood for sexual intercourse. It can also be used as a sort of fun and intimate game of taking turns. You and your partner can take turns performing oral sex on one another and bring each other close to climax before stopping and doing it all over again. See how many turns each of you can take before you need to give in to the release of your desire.

8. Be open and respectful both as the giver and the receiver. Share with your partner what you are comfortable with regarding ejaculation before performing oral sex. If you need them to warn you so you can change positions, that is okay. Communicate in order to understand each other's needs and comfort levels.

9. Have fun and be creative as you explore your partner's body. Do not worry about orgasm as an end goal. Be present and in the moment in order to create an environment that leads to relaxation, arousal, and pure enjoyment.

Oral Sex Positions

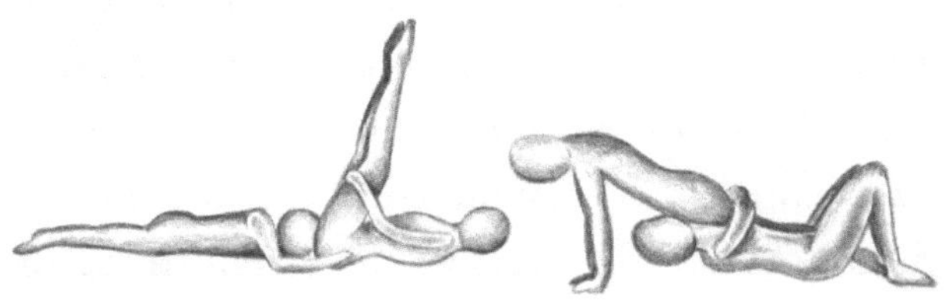

A. Gorge   B. Deep Throat

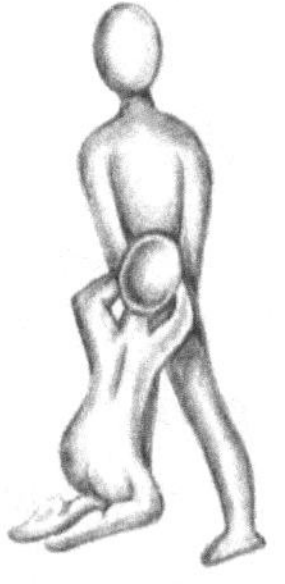
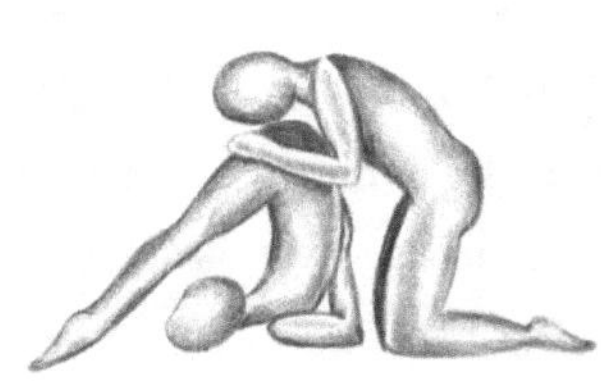

C. Zeus   D. Pisces

A. **The Gorge:** The receiving partner lies comfortably on their back with their head on a pillow and their legs bent together and lifted up in a vertical position. The penetrating partner sits on their knees or lies flat in front of the receiving partner, facing their genitalia.

B. **Deep Throat:** This position puts the receiving partner's head at the ultimate angle for deep throat penetration. The receiving partner leans back against a couch, chair, or bed with pillows. The penetrating partner can achieve this angle from a kneeling, squatting, or standing position.

          WHERE INTIMACY BEGINS

C. **Zeus:** The penetrating partner stands with their legs at shoulder width; the receiving/giving partner stands on their knees in front, facing their partner's genital area. The penetrating partner can take the giving partner's head to control the rhythm; the other hugs the buttocks and proceeds with the process.

D. **Pisces:** The giving partner sits on their feet. The receiving partner lies down on the giving partner's knees with their head and shoulders on the floor; legs are straight, slightly driven apart, and half pressed to the body. The giving partner leans forward so their face is between the receiving partner's legs.

Mutual pleasure is key when it comes to enjoying oral sex. Great oral sex results from knowing what your partner wants and also communicating your own needs and desires. Effective communication between the giver and the receiver takes time and practice, but is definitely worth it. When you take the time to get to know your partner's body and explore what makes them feel good, you'll elevate your closeness and your bond.

Stage 10

━━━❧❧❧━━━

THE GRAND FINALE

The benefits of a healthy and creative sex life are endless. It can boost self-esteem, increase your ability to experience pleasure, and develop both emotional and physical intimacy with your partner. Sex, especially when climax is reached, can reduce stress, burn calories, improve your mood, boost your immune system, and help with sleep. Being sexually creative and open can promote a lasting and fulfilling intimate relationship.

Although orgasm is considered the peak of sexual arousal and results in a very intense and pleasurable feeling, it's not always the end goal. The sexual act in itself is the true bonding experience and climaxing is an added bonus for most. Orgasms can be reached through various creative and fun measures of foreplay, sexual intercourse, and/or masturbation. Everyone is different, and it is important to explore the ways in which you and your partner reach climax. For some women, receiving oral sex is an easier and more pleasurable way to orgasm. For others, manual stimulation does the trick. No matter what your preference, when orgasm is reached, our brains and bodies are flooded with feel-good hormones that promote bliss and bonding.

We encourage you to try something new in the bedroom with your partner. The loss of novelty when referring to sex can pose some challenges, so why not spice things up and experiment? You may discover a new pleasure point or a new approach that you'd like to explore. The addition of sex toys, blindfolds, wrist ties, and implementing role-play can elevate your sex life. Try a new position or change up the pace of sex. Hot and fast sex can be thrilling and fun, but if that is your go-to, try slowing things down. Take time to feel your bodies moving in sync, and get into a rhythm that connects you both emotionally and physically.

Discover a new sexual position and have fun! Encourage each other to take risks, be vulnerable, and grow together through experimentation. We have included a few of our favorite sexual positions in the following diagram.

Sexual Positions

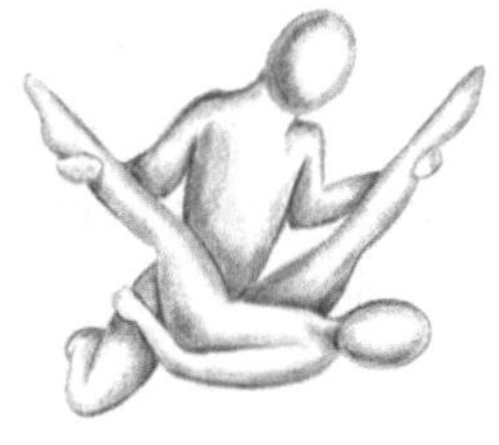

A. Captain

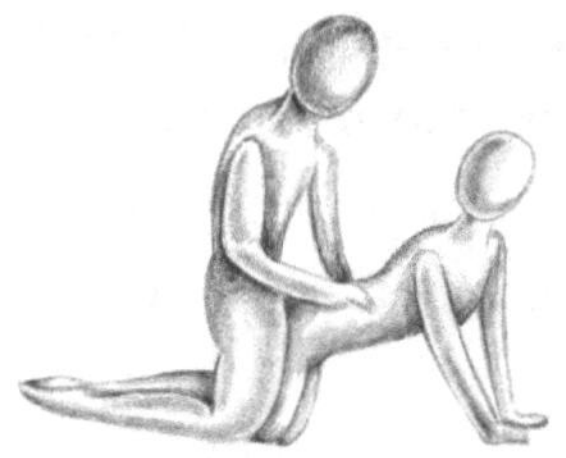

B. Doggy Style

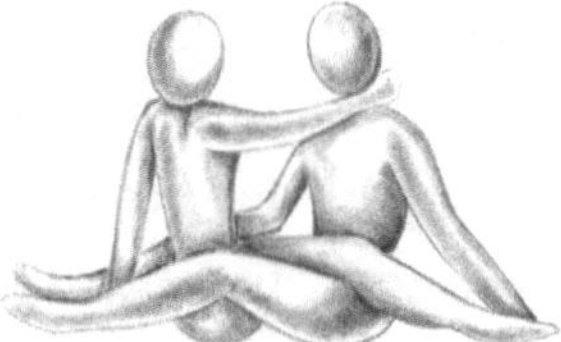

C. Straddle

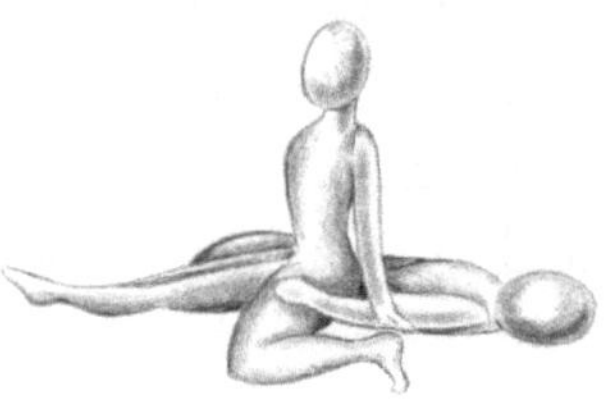

D. Reverse Cowgirl

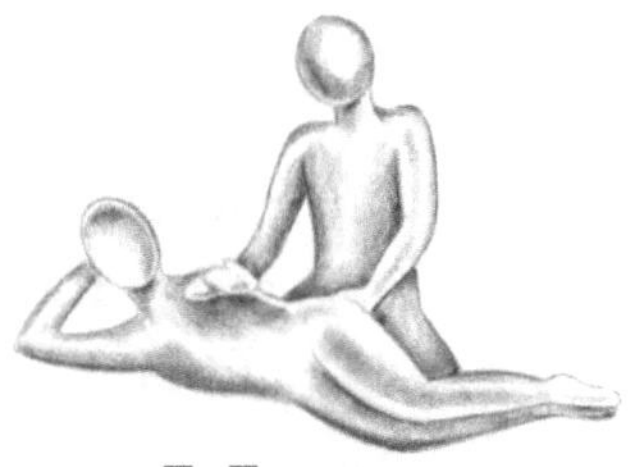

E. Emperor

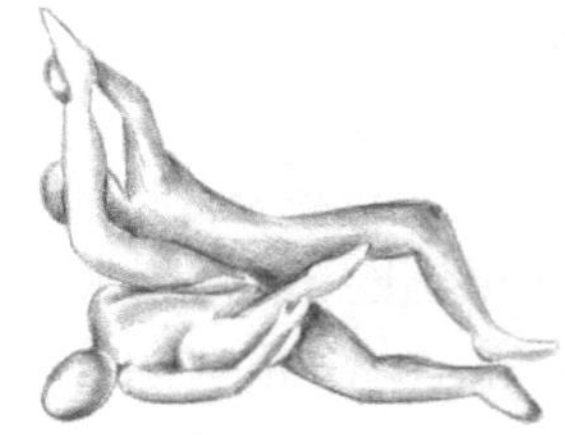

F. T-Square

A. **Captain:** The receiving partner lies on their back with their legs in the air or resting on their partner's shoulders while the penetrating partner kneels in front and inserts their penis or sex toy.

B. **Doggy Style:** The receiving partner gets on all fours while the penetrating partner kneels behind them and inserts their penis or sex toy into the vagina or anus.

   WHERE INTIMACY BEGINS

C. **Straddle:** The penetrating partner sits down facing the receiving partner. The receiving partner straddles the penetrating partner and inserts the penis or sex toy into the vagina or anus.

D. **Reverse Cowgirl:** The penetrating partner lies on their back while the receiving partner straddles them, facing their feet. The top partner can then bounce on, grind against, or "ride" the bottom partner's penis or sex toy.

E. **Emperor:** This is one of the many variations of the spoon or adjusted spoon position. The receiving partner lies on their side facing away from their partner, while the penetrating partner kneels behind them and inserts the penis or sex toy while performing a thrusting motion.

F. **T-Square:** To get into this position, the giver lies on their side, while the receiver lies perpendicular to them and raises their legs. After penetration, the receiver lowers their legs so their knees are bent over their partner's waist and thighs, or you can get creative and hold your legs back. This position is great when neither partner has an excess of stamina. It is also wonderful for clitoral stimulation if the receiving partner is female.

Sexual intercourse is an important and valued part of many romantic relationships. The level of your sexual activity depends on your personal taste, physical desires, and the status or nature of your relationship. The grand finale is not always about orgasm; the true climax is the continuing sexual experience you make and maintain with passion and purpose.

Appendix A

———〜〜〜———

The Great Climax

Cliff Notes for Stages 1 through 10

Stage 1: Get naked, loosen up, and know your own body. How do you like to get off? Touch yourself and get comfortable with all of your parts. **LOVE YOURSELF.**

Stage 2: Shut your phone off, talk to your partner, and tune in to them. **LISTEN.**

Stage 3: Spend some **TIME** together and do it often without distractions. Go on **DATES**.

Stage 4: Be **NICE.** No one wants to fuck a dick; well, you know what we mean.

Stage 5: Know your partner's **LOVE LANGUAGE** and your own. You may have to go back and review this topic if you are unsure of what that means.

Stage 6: Be **OPEN**, explore, and push your boundaries; there are several ways to climax. How do you know what you like if you've never tried it?

Stage 7: Have some **FUN. FLIRT** with your partner or become someone else for the night. Don't forget to **PLAY.**

Stage 8: Engage all the **SENSES.** Your orgasm can be bigger than even you realize.

Stage 9: Grabbing their bits as the only form of **FOREPLAY** doesn't count. Go back and read if this speaks to you. **PLEASURE** your partner. **ORAL SEX** can be wonderful.

Stage 10: Orgasm is not always the end goal. Enjoy the build-up. Enjoy the process. **ENJOY EACH OTHER**.

The Box is waiting; go find your Bond.

Appendix B

<hr>

EMOTIONAL INTIMACY EXERCISES

I. BODY AFFIRMATIONS (SOLO OR AS A COUPLE)

1. Stand up straight in a comfortable place wearing only your underwear.
2. Close your eyes and picture your body naked.
3. Remind yourself how lucky you are to have this beautiful body.
4. Repeat (with your eyes still closed), "I am beautiful. I am brave. I am grateful for my body. I respect my body. This body gives me the opportunity to enjoy such an amazing experience. I am beautiful. I love my body."
5. Open your eyes and tell yourself this again as you look in the mirror. Smile as you start this new adventure of self-love.

II. Getting to Know Your Desires Activity

Take some time to get to know yourself and your partner better. Ask some questions. Here are a few to get started:

1. Which genre of music do you like and what emotions does it elicit? Music can influence your mood and can be a useful tool in self-discovery.
2. Do you like to be touched softly or does it tickle? Do you prefer it hard?
3. Do you like having a certain body part touched or massaged? Be specific.
4. Where do you like to be kissed? Share your preferences.
5. What types of fantasies are you okay with exploring? Open up about your desires.
6. What are some fantasies you are not comfortable exploring? It's good to share both.

If you are having difficulty coming up with your own questions, try conversation cards.

You can also journal these ideas for self exploration to better understand yourself prior to sharing with a partner.

Appendix C

PHYSICAL TOUCH SUGGESTIONS

Eye gazing: Look into each other's eyes. Feel the energy that is exchanged during this activity. What are you feeling, remembering, or desiring? What do you think your partner is experiencing while looking back at you?

Smiling: Show your partner that you're happy to see them and be with them through a simple smile while looking directly at them.

Physical closeness: Stand close to each other and feel the warmth of the skin. Lean against your partner's body. Feel the energy between you.

Light touch: Lightly touch and caress one another. This can be done while in bed or relaxing on the couch. Touch your partner's limbs, neck, face, head (play with their hair). Lightly run your fingers down your partner's back.

Hugging: Soft hugs and holding your partner offer safety and support. Smell each other; feel each other's heart beat. Hug your partner when they are feeling down to offer encouragement and love.

Cuddling: Holding and snuggling with your partner while in bed or on the couch can be very satisfying while providing a sense of comfort and can increase your sense of security.

Massages: Giving your partner a neck, shoulder, back, or full body massage is an excellent way to connect and relax. It can easily lead to arousal and an intimate experience if that is your desire. Use lotions or oils to elevate the experience.

Kissing: Small kisses in tender places can be a form of foreplay. Kissing each other when you greet or are going to sleep can speak someone's love language. Deep passionate kisses when heating things up can increase the intensity of your sexual experience. Use your tongue when it feels right.

Nipple stimulation: The nipples are very sensitive for both men and women. Engaging in nipple play by massaging, flicking, pinching, tugging, and licking can be very erotic and increase intensity of arousal. There are many different types of oils, stimulators, and vibrating toys that can be used for additional nipple stimulation. For some, nipple orgasms are possible.

Vaginal stimulation*: Fingering is a technique typically using your first and/or middle fingers. Start slowly by entering one to two fingers into the vulva. Slowly open the vulva and gently touch the clitoris. Before you dip into the vagina, turn your partner on by touching the exterior anatomy which is very sensitive to arousal. Run gentle circles in areas where they feel most aroused. Moving into the vagina, use gentle pressure on the G-spot. This is an area inside and close to the vaginal opening that feels spongy and firm. Then increase the pressure and movement to heighten arousal. Lubrication is recommended. Oral stimulation can be extremely erotic. Be sure to refer back to Stage 8: Exploring Oral for specific guidelines in this area. Vibrators offer great options for vaginal stimulation as well.

Penile stimulation*: The "hand job" is touching the penis, best done with lubrication. Start gently and apply pressure as you go. The base of the shaft tolerates firm pressure better than the tip. This area (the head/glans) is the most sensitive, and pressure tolerances are very individual. Slide your hand up and down with rhythmic movements. Cupping your hand and rolling it around the head of the penis can be very arousing. Pay careful attention to what your partner is telling you they like both verbally and with their body language. Vibrator use can also be arousing.

Taint stimulation: The taint is the perineum or area between genitals and anus. Gently lick, massage, or vibrate this area for increased sexual arousal.

Anal stimulation*: This is a no-go zone for some. For those willing to explore, start gently with pressure on the anus. Lubrication is recommended. You may advance to using fingers, toys, vibrators, and genitals for penetration as tolerated.

***See Appendix D: A Lesson in Sexual Anatomy**

A LESSON IN SEXUAL ANATOMY

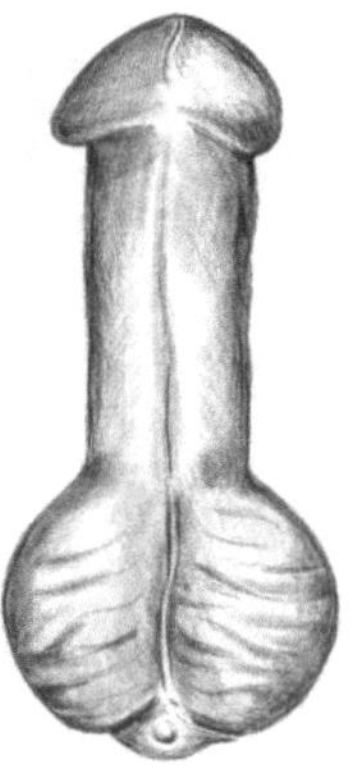 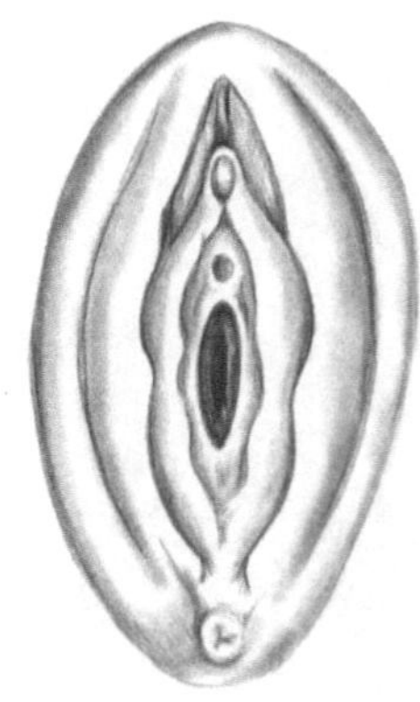

Penis	Vagina
Urethra—The tube that carries urine out of the bladder and also transports semen from the ejaculatory ducts.	**Mons Pubis**—The mound of fatty tissue over the pubic bone.
Head (glans)—A sensitive area where the urethra is located.	**Vulva**—The outer part made up of the labia majora, labia minora, and clitoris.
Frenulum—A small tag of skin on the underside of the penis between the foreskin and shaft.	**Labia Majora**—The larger, fleshy lips of tissue that enclose and protect the other external entities.

<table>
<tr>
<td>

Shaft—The shaft of the penis extends from the tip or head to the base.

Scrotum (or scrotal sac)—A part of the external male genitalia located behind and underneath the penis. Houses the testicles.

Anus—Posterior opening of the digestive tract.

</td>
<td>

Labia Minora—The smaller lips inside the labia majora.

Clitoris—A small overhang that is highly sensitive to sexual stimulation and can become erect.

Urethral Opening—Area in which urine from the bladder meets the outside.

Perineum—The perineum (taint) is the area between the genitals and anus.

Vaginal Opening—This area is between the perineum and urethral opening.

Anus—Posterior opening of the digestive tract.

</td>
</tr>
</table>

Appendix E

<hr>

PLAY ACTIVITIES

ROLE-PLAY SUGGESTION

Massage Therapist and Client

When I got home this evening and opened my front door, soft music and candlelight filled the room and my partner was waiting for me. They* greeted me with a smile, took my bag, and handed me a plush white robe. They were dressed in scrubs, their hair pulled back tightly, and their hands had been recently moisturized. The smell of lavender and eucalyptus was in the air and reminded me of a spa that we had visited in the past.

I went into the bathroom, undressed, and put on the robe. When I walked out of the bathroom, they escorted me to a mat on the floor with a soft blanket on top. They told me to lie down, take off my robe, and pull a blanket over my body. I did as they requested, and they pulled down the blanket and began rubbing warm oil all over my back, buttocks, and legs. They then started to ask me how it felt—if I would like it harder or softer, if I wanted to turn over. They started talking dirty to me while massaging me and began kissing my neck and my ear. They started teasing me with soft kisses then hard massage, while whispering naughty phrases. Then suddenly they stopped and resumed character.

They told me to turn over, then put my wrists together and tied my hands together. They began massaging my pelvic area, started kissing my thighs and licking my toes. I started feeling a hot and tingly feeling all over my body. I didn't want this to stop. After many moments just like this, they started to give me oral pleasure. My release was incredible under their careful touch. It was their turn next.

This can be played to your own preferences while taking turns.

*"They" is used because the dominant and submissive roles can be played by either partner at any time.

ADDITIONAL PLAY ACTIVITIES

A Game of Hide and Seek

Taking this childhood game to another level with your partner is a novel and fun way to connect and laugh. It is also a great way to practice your foreplay skills.

- Wear comfy or sexy clothes.
- Turn the lights down, burn candles, and/or in the dark.

- One person closes their eyes and counts to twenty-five, giving their partner time to find a place to hide.
- The seeker tries to find the hider. And then take turns.
- Whoever finds the hider gets to take off a piece of the other's clothing or ask for one sexual favor for ten seconds.
- Take turns and heighten your desire by teasing your partner as you continue to play.

Body Paint Foreplay

Body painting can be a fun and sexual experience that you both enjoy. Stop by your local adult shop or browse online to pick an edible body paint.

- Be sure to grab towels and/or wipes for cleanup later.
- If you have a blow-up mattress, it might be a good idea to use that. If not, cover your surface with sheets and/or towels.
- Choose a tool to paint your partner's body (paintbrush, feather, flower, fingertips, tongue).
- Think about a design before you begin. Take your time; don't rush to the hot spots immediately. Ease into them, tease your partner, build up the anticipation and arousal.
- Try a blindfold or glow-in-the-dark paint to change it up for the next time.

Food Play

Mixing food and sex is an easy and delicious way to spice up your sex life.

- Create a clean space that you can lie down on and use edible items nearby. (The kitchen table is a great place.)
- Choose one or more edible items that you both enjoy (strawberries, whipped cream, chocolate syrup, etc.).
- One partner lies down naked or in lingerie/undies.
- The other partner places drips or lathers a body part (breasts, stomach, inner thighs, etc.) with the food item.
- Explore textures and temperatures. Discuss what you like and don't like.
- This foreplay may lead you to the shower. You can then switch roles and have some more fun.

Final Thoughts

Hopefully, as you have experienced this journey, you have learned a little, laughed a lot, and now find yourself enveloped in love. You are on a path of forever strengthening and lengthening your bond. The deep connection you are cultivating will help carry you through the many seasons of your relationship. The goal is for your bond to be unbreakable.

We would like to take a moment to recognize that these intimacy tips, suggestions, or activities may not be for everyone. If you find yourself or your partner suffering from any physical or emotional discomfort during this experience, there are professional services that may be helpful. Don't be afraid to reach out to your local gynecologist, sex therapist, or psychologist for additional guidance and support if you feel you may need it.

At our core, we are passionate about connection, and we maintain our commitment to bringing you novel ideas and guidance for fostering intimacy. Visit us at TheBondedBox.com for our latest drops and custom experiences as you continue on your journey.

A sincere thank you for joining us and prioritizing your bond in a world that struggles to slow down to connect. Until the next time, continue to vibe high and share your love.

Affectionately yours,
The Founders